Surviving Prostate Cancer/Cook Book

Vegan Cook Book Contents

I0422954

Surviving Prostate Cancer

Chapter 1

In 1991 I was 51 years old, self employed and busting my butt trying to keep my head above water. I was suffering with a severe cold that I was having a difficult time getting rid of. The doctor I elected to see was recommended by a friend as I did not have a primary care physician. He asked me if I had had a PSA (prostate-specific antigen) test lately. I replied no. Thinking back on this time I'm not sure if I even knew what that was, but blood was draw and at some later date he informed me that my PSA was slightly elevated but nothing to worry about and that we would check it again next time I came to see him. I never had it checked again for 12 years. What a bonehead.

The [1] PSA, prostate-specific antigen test measures an enzyme produced almost exclusively by the glandular cells of the prostate. It is secreted during ejaculation into the prostatic ducts that empty into the urethra. PSA liquefies semen after ejaculation, promoting the release of sperm.

Normally, only very small amounts of PSA are present in the blood. But an abnormality of the prostate can disrupt the normal architecture of the gland and create an opening for PSA to pass into the bloodstream. Thus, high blood levels of PSA can indicate prostate problems, including cancer.

Now, research reported in *BMC Medicine* (Volume 6, page 6), indicates that a man's prostate-specific antigen (PSA) level at or before age 50 can predict his risk of developing advanced prostate cancer 25 years later.

Researcher's analyzed data from blood samples collected from about 21,000 men between 1974 and 1986 as part of the Malmö [Sweden] Preventive Medicine Study. By 1999, 498 of the men had developed prostate cancer. Because not all elevated PSA levels indicate a clinically relevant cancer, the researchers focused only on the risk of developing locally advanced or metastatic prostate cancer. This was defined as the presence of metastases or as clinical stage T3 or higher at the time of diagnosis. By this definition, 161 of the men had potentially life-threatening disease.

Bottom line: The researchers found that a man's PSA level around age 50 was a strong predictor of the development of advanced prostate cancer later in life. Even a modestly increased PSA level, 1.01 to 2.0 ng/mL, increased the odds of developing advanced prostate cancer by several percentage points. *These results suggest that PSA levels in middle age might be used to determine which men need more intensive prostate cancer screening and which can be screened less frequently.*

What age is too old for annual PSA testing? Well, according to the USPSTF (U.S. Preventive Services Task Force) men 75 and older should no longer be screened. The potential benefits and harms of PSA testing in this population screening were more likely to have a negative impact on these men than a positive one.

Since most prostate cancer is a slow-growing malignancy, that may take 10 or more years to produce significant symptoms, many elderly men will die of another condition before their prostate cancer becomes life threatening. Thus, an abnormal PSA test would lead to the pain and discomfort of a prostate biopsy and unnecessary worry if no cancer is found. If cancer is found and treated, the man will have to contend with side effects, such as sexual dysfunction and incontinence.

Other medical organizations recommend annual screening for men at average risk for prostate cancer beginning at age 50, but they do not address when screening is no longer necessary. And still others recommend screening for all men with a life expectancy of at least 10 years.

If you are age 75 or older, discuss the risks and benefits of PSA testing with your doctor. If you get tested and are diagnosed with a low-grade cancer, keep in mind that active surveillance is an option that allows you to be closely monitored but treated only if your disease progresses.

Several years after I had my PSA test I slipped and fell at my warehouse and landed on the left side of my left knee. I couldn't straighten that leg. I called a few local doctors until I found one who could see me right away. They took an x-ray and found that a chunk of calcium build-up had broken off and was wedged in the knee joint. He recommended surgery. I owned my own business and was my only employee and surgery was financially out of the question yet I couldn't work as I drove a van delivering supplies. Miss a day and I was in trouble financially. I called a friend of mine who is a pediatric surgeon, told him my problem, and asked how much this was going to cost me. He said he would do the surgery for nothing but that the hospital would charge about 5K. Once again out of my budget and I also would be laid up for awhile. So I called my mother and asked if she could come over and help me with a garage sale so I could raise enough for the surgery and cover the days I would lose income. She said to me, "Why don't you go to the VA? You're a veteran". I slapped my forehead like on the V8 commercial and thought why didn't I think of that. Since I couldn't drive she came over and drove me to the VA. They gave me a shot of cortisone and I was able to straighten my leg. The doctor told me I would probably need another cortisone shot at some future date and possible surgery sometime thereafter. It was about this time that I started taking vitamin supplements from a company called USANA. One of the supplements was **Procosa® II**. **Procosa® II** is not only an excellent source of glucosamine; it's formulated with vitamin C, manganese, and silicon to provide additional nutrition essential for optimal joint health. Another advantage of Procosa II is that it contains turmeric extract, speeding the supplement's action to provide more immediate benefits. I've never had another problem with that knee since. What has this to do with my prostate cancer? Well, nothing really, but it got me going to the VA for checkups on a more regular basis. Thank God... and my mom. Not necessarily in that order mom.

I would like to give you a little background on USANA because I feel it has had a marked effect on my cancer recovery. [2]Dr. Myron

Wentz, internationally recognized microbiologist, immunologist, and pioneer in the development of human cell culture technology and infectious disease diagnoses, holds a bachelor's degree in biology from North Central College in Naperville, Illinois, a master's degree in microbiology from the University of North Dakota, and a Ph.D. in microbiology and immunology from the University of Utah in Salt Lake City.

Joining a pathology group in Peoria, Illinois, Dr. Wentz served as infectious diseases specialist and directed the microbiology and immunology laboratories for three hospitals in the Peoria area. After three years of clinical experience, he saw an opportunity to make a deeper contribution to medical science by developing much-needed tests for viral diseases.

Dr. Wentz launched Gull Laboratories as a one-man operation in 1974. By June of 1977, several of his viral diagnostic assays were FDA-approved and ready for marketing to hospitals and clinical laboratories. He developed the first commercially available test for diagnosing infection with the Epstein-Barr virus. Dr. Wentz sold his controlling interests in Gull Laboratories in 1992 and founded USANA Health Sciences, a state-of-the-art manufacturer of nutritional supplements, foods, and personal-care products.

Even though his businesses have been extremely successful, Dr. Wentz first and foremost considers himself to be a scientist, not a businessman. Nonetheless, Dr. Wentz' business acumen has been recognized through a presidential appointment as an advisor to the Small Business Administration and as a 2003 recipient of the Utah Ernst & Young Entrepreneur of the Year award.

In addition to Gull Laboratories and USANA Health Sciences, Dr. Wentz created Sanoviv Medical Institute, a holistic medical facility with full hospital accreditation located in Baja California. In recent years Dr. Wentz has turned his attention to charitable and humanitarian concerns, founding the Wentz Medical Centre and Laboratory in Uganda and the Wentz Medical Centre in Cambodia to serve children in those countries orphaned by diseases such as malaria and HIV. In 2006 Dr. Wentz was a recipient of the

Children's Champion Award, presented by the Children's Hunger Fund, for which he travels worldwide as a medical missionary. In 2007 Dr. Wentz was honored with the Albert Einstein Award for Outstanding Achievement in the Life Sciences. In the final analysis, it is his dream to help people live longer healthier lives, that drives Dr. Wentz so relentlessly. Such a pace could be attributed to an unusually high level of energy. But Dr. Wentz attributes it to something else: an urgent sense of mission. "I have always felt that the time is too short for me, that life is too short for what I feel I need to get done," he says. "I was too late to help my father. I was too late to help my mother. But I think I am making contributions that are now allowing people to live the way they were intended to live: in health. I think I am helping people live their lives to the fullest without having them cut short by premature death or illness." Do yourself a favor and investigate for yourself the USANA story. It is more important now than ever before to supplement your diet. I'll tell you why a little later.

Chapter 2

In the early part of 2003 I noticed I had blood in my semen. I went to the VA and was told this was normal... NORMAL! Well I was stupid enough to listen to the doctor tell me that at my age this was a common occurrence. So I went on my merry way.

In October of the same year I went for a physical and to have a sigmoidoscopy. My NEW doctor asked me if I had ever had a DRE... the dreaded digital rectal exam. Ah, no! I replied. Where upon she slipped on a pair of surgical gloves and told me to assume the position. She told me that she felt some hard lumps during the exam and wanted to have blood drawn for a PSA test. Two weeks later she called and asked me to come in. She sat me down and informed me that I had prostate cancer and that my PSA score was 121. I had no clue as to what that meant. I simply asked, "What do we do now? She replied that they had a doctor who worked at the UCLA prostate cancer research center that came to the VA one day a week and that she would make an appointment for me to have blood drawn again a week before seeing him. The fact that he only came 1 day a week meant that it would be about 30 days before I could see him. Now here is the first step in surviving prostate cancer... don't panic and don't jump to a fatalistic attitude.

For the next 30 days I maintained a positive attitude thinking only about what it was that they were going to do to help conquer this problem. I don't remember thinking once about dying. I arrived at the VA at the appointed time and waited to see the doctor. The waiting room was about half full of what I assumed were all prostate cancer patients. Presently I was called and placed in a room to wait some more... military... hurry up and wait. Doctor Aronson, a young man of about 35 came in and introduced himself and said he would like to also give me a DRE... sadists, everyone of them. After the exam he entered a few lines in the computer and then turned to me and informed me that there are two types of prostate cancer, slow growing and aggressive. I had the latter. My score was now 161.... 40 points in less than 30 days, 20 days actually. Now remember, step 1? Don't panic? I didn't panic. The next step was a biopsy as the PSA test is only an indicator of possible cancer. If you've never had a biopsy on your prostate gland it feels like when you were a little kid and your sister pinched you real hard on the arm… remember how that felt? Depending upon your age it probably made you cry. Well it's kind of like that, but not too bad.

For a prostate biopsy [3], a thin needle is inserted through the rectum (transrectal biopsy), through the urethra, or through the area between the anus and scrotum (perineum). A transrectal biopsy is the most common method used. Prior to the biopsy, they put you on a mega dose of anti-biotic, and the day before you fast and drink a colon flush. The tissue samples taken during the biopsy are examined for cancer cells. The method used to perform the biopsy in my case was the transrectal method. Four samples were taken from each side of the prostate gland which resembles a walnut. The results of the biopsy are scored from 0 – 10 on the Gleason Score [4]. The Gleason score was invented in 1966 by Dr. Donald Gleason, a pathologist. He based the score on information derived from studies of the biopsies of nearly 3,000 patients who had been diagnosed with prostate cancer. Pathologists worldwide rely on the Gleason score. The score provides an effective measurement that helps your doctor determine how severe your prostate cancer is, based on the appearance of the cancer cells when viewed under a microscope. All cancer looks abnormal to a pathologist, but low-grade cancers have cells that often look similar to healthy cells from the gland or organ that has been affected by the cancer. As a result, the pathologist can recognize that she's looking at prostate cells under the microscope. But when the cancer is aggressive, the cancer cells look less and less like normal prostate cells (or any other kind of cells). Pathologists find the Gleason grading system to be very reliable. For example, if the Gleason score indicates that the cancer is an intermediate risk cancer (a Gleason score of 7) it nearly always *is* an intermediate risk. As a result, doctors can make predictions from Gleason grades. The more distorted and aggressive the cancer looks, the higher the Gleason grade, and the more aggressive the cancer behaves in the body. My score… 8.

He proceeded to tell me that he was putting me on hormone treatments, a shot every 3 months of Zoladex. [5] Zoladex is used to treat advanced prostate cancer. These medicines block the production of testosterone. The procedure is often called chemical castration, because it has the same result as surgical removal of the testes. However, unlike surgery, it is reversible. The drugs must be given by injection, usually every 3 - 6 months. Possible side effects include nausea and vomiting, hot flashes, anemia, lethargy, osteoporosis, reduced sexual desire, and impotence. I had several of those symptoms, hot flashes being the worst along with reduced sexual desire. I was, and still am, single, and wasn't dating anyone at the time, so reduced sexual desire was not a problem. Hot flashes and mood swings... another matter altogether. I would awake in the middle of the night drenched in sweat only to awake later freezing cold as I had opened the window. This was in the dead of winter. Good timing.

The Zoladex injection is given in the abdominal area, just under the skin. They spray the area with a numbing compound then insert a needle about the size of a torpedo under the skin and plunge the plunger. Actually it's not so bad unless you get the nurse from hell, which I did ONCE. She slowly pushed the needle, which is actually the size of maybe two pencil leads, into my stomach fat. They go straight in until they puncture the skin and then turn the needle parallel to your stomach then inject the Zoladex. It looks like a small, long thin capsule about an inch in length. She kept pushing until she had made a dent in my stomach of about an inch before she punctured my flesh. I made it abundantly clear to the receptionist afterwards that I was to never see her again. Nurse Rachett was a sadist. Now for a little technical jargon:

According to the American Cancer Society, hormone therapy [6] may be used in several situations:

- if you are not able to have surgery or radiation or can't be cured by these treatments because the cancer has already spread beyond the prostate gland

- if your cancer remains or comes back after treatment with surgery or radiation therapy

- as an addition to radiation therapy as initial treatment if you
  are at high risk for cancer recurrence

- before surgery or radiation to try and shrink the cancer to
  make other treatments more effective

Hormone therapy is also called androgen deprivation therapy (ADT)
or androgen suppression therapy. The goal is to reduce levels of the
male hormones, called androgens, in the body. The main androgens
are testosterone and dihydrotestosterone (DHT). Androgens,
produced mainly in the testicles, stimulate prostate cancer cells to
grow. Lowering androgen levels often makes prostate cancers shrink
or grow more slowly. However, hormone therapy does not cure
prostate cancer.

There are several types of hormone therapy used to treat prostate
cancer.

- Orchiectomy (surgical castration)
- Luteinizing hormone-releasing hormone (LHRH) agonist
- Luteinizing hormone-releasing hormone (LHRH) antagonists
- Anti-androgens
- Other androgen-suppressing drugs

Goserelin acetate (Zoladex, AstraZeneca) is an injectable
gonadotropin releasing hormone super-agonist (GnRH agonist), also
known as a lutenizing hormone releasing hormone (LHRH) agonist.
Goserelin acetate is used to suppress production of the sex hormones
(testosterone and estrogen), particularly in the treatment of breast
and prostate cancer.

In biochemistry, agonists are compounds that stimulate the
production of another compound. (In contrast, antagonists are
compounds that suppress the production of another compound.)
Goserelin acetate stimulates the production of the sex hormones
testosterone and estrogen. However, these hormones are regulated by
feedback loops. So paradoxically, after goserelin stimulates the
production of sex hormones, the hormones are then suppressed by
the body's feedback mechanisms.

Prostate cancer cells and some breast cancer cells are hormone-dependent, that is, they need hormone stimulation to grow. When the hormones are eliminated, the cancer cells are inhibited.

Zoladex was approved by the U.S. Food and Drug Administration in 1989 for treatment of prostate cancer. Other indications were subsequently approved.

Goserelin is a hormone similar to the one normally released from the hypothalamus gland in the brain. It is used to treat a number of medical problems. These include:

- Cancer of the prostate in men
- Cancer of the breast in women if it develops before or around the time of menopause
- Endometriosis, a painful condition caused by extra tissue growing inside or outside of the uterus, and
- Thinning of the lining of the uterus before surgery on the uterus.

When given regularly as an implant, goserelin works every day to decrease the amount of estrogen and testosterone in the blood.

Goserelin is poorly protein bound and has a serum elimination half-life of two to four hours in patients with normal renal function. The half-life increases with patients with impaired renal function. There is no significant change in pharmacokinetics in subjects with hepatic failure. After administration, peak serum concentrations are reached in about two hours. It rapidly binds to the LHRH receptor cells in the pituitary gland thus leading to an initial increase in production of luteinizing hormone and thus leading to an initial increase in the production of corresponding sex hormones. This initial Flare may be treated by co-prescribing/co-administering Casodex (Bicalutamide) or similar medication. Eventually, after a period of about 14–21 days, production of LH is greatly reduced due to receptor down regulation, and sex hormones are generally reduced to castrate levels.

There are side effects to hormone therapy as I stated previously:

- Reduced or absent libido (sexual desire). *Ah, yep.*
- Impotence. *Oh yeah.*
- Hot flashes (these may get better or even go away with time). *I had them after I was off therapy for a year. Not as intense, but still there.*
- Breast tenderness and growth of breast tissue. *Yep again.*
- Osteoporosis (bone thinning), which can lead to broken bones.
- Anemia (low red blood cell counts).
- Decreased mental acuity (sharpness). *Duh, not sure about that one, I AM 70.*
- Loss of muscle mass. *That 70 thing again.*
- Weight gain. *20 pounds, still have it after being off Zoladex for 2 years.*
- Fatigue. *70 again… who knows.*
- Increased cholesterol. *Yes! But under control.*
- Depression. *Well no kidding… I have cancer.*

With all that said I was put on quarterly injections of Zoladex. Let the hot flashes begin.

For those of you who are concerned about the increase in body fat and absence of libido there has been some talk about taking testosterone supplements… fugetaboutit, I have no need for testosterone. I mean I'm trying to eliminate it. You have no guarantee of the safety or effectiveness of any dietary supplement, including those promoted as natural hormones. Dietary supplements do not have to undergo the rigorous testing that pharmaceuticals do. This statement may seem contrary to what I mentioned about supplementation so I encourage you to do your due diligence, especially about USANA.

There are potential dangers in the use of unregulated supplements. The University of Texas Southwestern Medical Center in Dallas reported that two men, both within the age of 50 to 70, developed metastatic prostate cancer within months of beginning a testosterone dietary supplement that was advertised in a fitness magazine. Both men had been screened for prostate cancer within the previous 11 months and were found to have normal PSA levels and digital rectal exams at that time.

While it's not possible to draw firm conclusions that the testosterone supplement was responsible for the cancer, laboratory experiments showed that it is a potent stimulator of prostate cancer cells. In addition, it made the cells resistant to the antiandrogen therapy used to treat advanced prostate cancer.

Johns Hopkins, in their Health Alerts [9], has mentioned a treatment. High-intensity focused ultrasound, or HIFU (pronounced HIGH-foo), is a promising technology for noninvasive tumor ablation that heats cancerous prostate tumors to near-boiling temperatures. Its *potential* clinical impact is indeed significant. But given the lack of long-term clinical data, Johns Hopkins advises caution.

"HIFU is the next frontier in prostate treatment," said John C. Rewcastle, Ph.D., Adjunct Assistant Professor of Radiology at The University of Calgary and medical director of EDAP, a manufacturer of Ablatherm, a HIFU device. Dr. Rewcastle is directing ongoing HIFU prostate cancer studies in Europe and the United States. "HIFU has the ability to answer the over-diagnosis and over-treatment questions that now surround prostate cancer treatment."

There are currently two HIFU devices for the treatment of prostate cancer: Sonablate (Focus Surgery, Inc., Indianapolis, Indiana) and Ablatherm (EDAP, Lyon, France). Although both devices are approved in Europe, Mexico, Canada, and the Far East, they are available in the U.S. for prostate cancer treatment only as part of ongoing Phase II/III trials to assess their safety and efficacy.

The Johns Hopkins Health Alert also states that age, race, and family history are important risk factors for prostate cancer. Diet and lifestyle factors may also be a factor in whether a man develops the disease. It has not been shown that there is an association in the development of prostate cancer and smoking, vasectomy, the presence of benign prostatic hyperplasia (BPH), regular alcohol intake, but binge drinking may increase the risk. Increasing evidence suggests that fat intake, physical inactivity, or being overweight may also influence the development or progression of prostate cancer.

Today watchful waiting for prostate cancer is most often recommended for men with low-grade prostate cancer that is believed to be small volume, especially older men whose prostate cancer is unlikely to become life threatening during their remaining years of life.

Men who choose watchful waiting must see their doctor regularly and undergo testing to determine whether the cancer is progressing. Recommendations on the frequency of visits and the tests conducted each time vary from doctor to doctor. Johns Hopkins recommends the following guidelines for men age 75 and younger who are in otherwise good health: PSA testing and a digital rectal exam twice a year and transrectal ultrasound and prostate biopsy once a year. The recommendations for PSA testing and digital rectal exams remain the same after age 75, but yearly ultrasound and prostate biopsy are no longer routinely performed.

Symptoms of Prostate Cancer

- Frequent or urgent need to urinate; delayed or interrupted urinary stream; dribbling.
- Pain upon urination.
- Blood in the urine.
- Painful or bloody ejaculation.
- Erectile dysfunction (impotence).
- Pain in the pelvis or lower back.

My only symptom was blood in my ejaculation as I stated earlier. And it was diagnosed as hematospermia. It can be a very alarming symptom. However, the good news is that bloody semen is almost never a sign of a serious underlying medical problem. Not in my case however, considering the fact that it wasn't that long afterwards that I was diagnosed with prostate cancer. I should have had a second opinion when I first noticed this and was told "it is normal". The fact that my PSA jumped 40 points in 20 days could have meant that if the hematospermia diagnosis had sent up an alarm at that time maybe my PSA score would have been significantly lower.

Possible sources for blood in the semen include the following:

- Urinary tract infections
- Prostatitis
- Sexually transmitted diseases such as gonorrhea or Chlamydia
- Benign prostate hypertrophy
- Surgical procedures such as prostate biopsy or bladder catheterization
- Trauma to the testicles or prostate
- Cancer of the prostate, bladder or reproductive organs

This now brings me to step 2. Share. Talk about your cancer, especially with your doctor. When someone asks about what you are doing about your cancer, tell them, even if they don't ask tell them anyway. It really helps to unburden yourself. Let it out. Give it to the universe as they say. And don't forget, it is always a good idea to get a second, third maybe even a fourth opinion on the treatment you decide upon.

Heart disease is the #1 killer of men, not prostate cancer, but research has shown that whatever is good for the health of your heart is also good for your prostate. When you take measures to protect your heart you are helping to counter the leading cause of early death while protecting your prostate, as well. If you can take your cardiac risk to zero, you will also be reducing your risk of prostate cancer to the lowest level possible.

The World Health Organization conducted a study in lifestyles and the researchers reported that a series of factors either caused a 90 to 95 percent reduction in heart attacks, or else explained 95 percent of the cardiac events they noted.

Nine factors that can help prevent heart attacks:

1. not smoking
2. low cholesterol (LDL less than 100 mg/dl)
3. good blood pressure (lower than 140 mmHg)
4. normal blood glucose
5. normal waist circumference: 36 inches or smaller
6. no depression
7. fruit and vegetable consumption with no limit
8. alcohol, in moderation; no more than two drinks a day
9. If aerobics is out of the question, walk for a minimum of 45 minutes daily.
   This last step will also help to maintain better bone mass and help prevent osteoporosis.

Chapter 3

The next step for me was to have a bone scan to determine if indeed the cancer had metastasized since my scores were so high. I arrived at the VA in Westwood, CA, and was sent directly to the basement where I was injected with a radioactive tracer substance into a vein in my arm. The tracer travels through the bloodstream and into the bones. This process may take several hours. A special camera (gamma) takes pictures of the tracer in the bones. This helps show cell activity and function in the bones. Areas that absorb little or no amount of tracer appear as dark or "cold" spots, which may indicate a lack of blood supply to the bone (bone infarction) or the presence of certain types of cancer. Areas of rapid bone growth or repair absorb increased amounts of the tracer and show up as bright or "hot" spots in the pictures. Hot spots may indicate problems such as arthritis, the presence of a tumor, a fracture, or an infection. After the injection I was told to come back in an hour to have the gamma pictures taken.

Thankfully the results were negative.

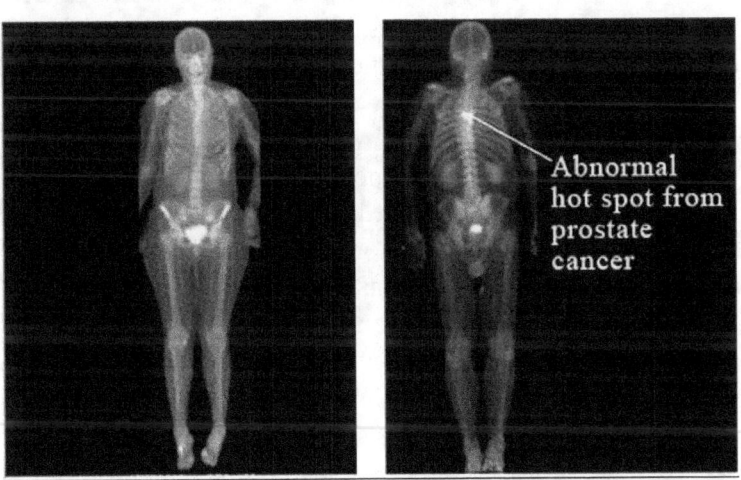

Abnormal hot spot from prostate cancer

[7] The first x-ray shows a normal scan of the prostate. The second is self explanatory.

My daughter Adrienne, who graduated from the USC Dental School and is now a dental hygienist, lived with a doctor and his wife while she was going to USC, Dr Waxman. Dr. Waxman, a neural surgeon, works at Cedar Sinai Hospital. Adrienne called him to make an appointment to get a second opinion. We spent about an hour with a Dr. Mitchell who looked at all my charts and x-rays and answered every question. He also wanted to give me a DRE. After he answered all our questions I said I had one more, "What are my chances of survival?" He said no problem you have at least 15 good years ahead. Now some irony for those of you who like irony... my grandfather died at 78 and my dad died at 78, and at this time I was 63. How's that for irony. But I'm going to beat the irony as well as the cancer.

There is another question men ask about prostate cancer and its causes. "If I have a vasectomy will I get prostate cancer"?

In March 1993, the [6]National Institute of Child Health and Human Development (NICHD) convened a conference, cosponsored by the National Cancer Institute (NCI) and the National Institute of Diabetes and Digestive and Kidney Diseases, to clarify the available evidence on the relationship between vasectomy and prostate cancer. Scientists reviewed and carefully weighed all of the data available at that time, including results from published and unpublished studies.

They determined that the results of research on the association between vasectomy and prostate cancer were not consistent. In addition, the scientists could not find any convincing biological explanation for a link between vasectomy and an increased risk of prostate cancer. Based on these findings, the expert panel concluded that even if having a vasectomy can increase a man's risk of developing prostate cancer, the increase in risk is relatively small.

In 1997, the NCI convened the prostate cancer Progress Review Group (PRG), a committee that included members from the scientific, medical, industrial, and advocacy communities. This group was charged with developing a national plan to outline scientific efforts involving prostate cancer research. The PRG's final report, published in August 1998, concluded that the evidence supporting a role for vasectomy in the development of prostate cancer is weak.

Researchers continue to investigate the possible relationship between vasectomy and prostate cancer. The majority of studies conducted thus far have upheld the conclusions made at the 1993 NICHD conference. Although a few studies have reported a link between vasectomy and prostate cancer, it is possible that other factors, including chance, may be responsible for the association suggested in these studies.

Chapter 4

During a follow up with my urologist, I asked him about radiation. He assured me that cancer research had shown that the hormone therapy was effective in fighting prostate cancer and that radiation, although it wouldn't hurt, wasn't necessary. Hey doc! Willy died, know what I mean? Several years later I had another opinion from a doctor who was visiting from Germany, he concurred with my doctor that radiation wasn't necessary. My daughter, God bless her, was more upset about this than I was. She said I needed to get radiation or else it would metastasize to my bones and I would die. Succinct and to the point wouldn't you say? She was very persistent... what can I say, she loves me. So I grabbed my cell and called her at work. I handed my doctor the phone after telling my daughter where I was. The man hardly uttered a word, not that he didn't try. After hanging up he handed me my phone and said... "Well, she's intense!" "You think?" I replied. So I opted for 40 radiation treatments.

The first step in my radiation therapy was to get a CT scan. This was to get the absolute critical positioning of my prostate. They place two small tattoos, one on each hip once the positioning is determined.

The doctor I met with at the VA prior to the radiation treatment, whose job it was to inform me about everything to expect during treatment, commented to me, "I don't know why you are wasting your time with radiation... I'm thinking, yeah I know the hormone therapy is adequate... your chances of survival are not good." I'm not sure now what I felt at that very moment, but after I got up to leave and was walking to my car, I broke down and the tears just flowed. Before I reached my car however, I stopped and said to myself, "Wait a minute, this guy isn't God. I'm going to beat this". I told my Urologist what he had said and when I went down for my first treatment this doctor's demeanor was entirely different... butter wouldn't melt in his mouth. He must have flunked bedside manner. Must have thought it was Bedside Manor and didn't want a room.

Radiation therapy [6] uses high-energy rays or particles to kill cancer cells. Radiation is sometimes used as the initial treatment for low-grade cancer that is still confined within the prostate gland or that has only spread to nearby tissue. Cure rates for men with these types of cancers are much like those for men getting radical prostatectomy (the surgical removal of the prostate gland). In the past prostatectomy was not a very viable solution as it damaged the nerves and erection became impossible. Now however, they have nerve sparing surgery that affords a very high chance of erectile function returning. Radiation is also sometimes used if the cancer is not completely removed or comes back (recurs) in the area of the prostate after surgery. If the disease is more advanced, radiation may be used to reduce the size of the tumor and to provide relief from present and possible future symptoms.

Two main types of radiation therapy are used: external beam radiation and brachytherapy (internal radiation). Both appear to be good methods of treating prostate cancer, although there is more long-term information about the results of treatment with external beam radiation.

The VA uses **Intensity modulated radiation therapy (IMRT):** IMRT is an advanced form of 3D therapy. It uses a computer-driven machine that actually moves around the patient as it delivers radiation. In addition to shaping the beams and aiming them at the prostate from several angles, the intensity (strength) of the beams can be adjusted to minimize the dose reaching the most sensitive normal tissues. This allows doctors to deliver an even higher dose to the cancer areas. Many major hospitals and cancer centers are now able to provide IMRT. The RapidArc™ is a form of IMRT that allows each treatment to be given over just a few minutes. It is more convenient for the patient, but is similar to regular IMRT in terms of effectiveness.

My treatments were every morning at 8am Monday thru Friday for 8 weeks or 40 treatments. It was a 30 minute drive in each direction. Each treatment lasted about 10 minutes from the time I lay down on the table till I got off the table. I believe they zapped me 5 times. Starting at about a 45 degree angle behind my hip to 45 in front of my hip to directly over my midsection and then to the 45's on the other side. At each position you could hear the machine making it's adjustments to the shape of my prostate in that position. That was it, thanks for coming see you tomorrow. There were supposed to be side effects from this as well:

- **Bowel problems:** During and after treatment with external beam radiation therapy, you may have diarrhea, sometimes with blood in the stool, rectal leakage, and an irritated large intestine. Most of these problems go away over time, but in rare cases normal bowel function does not return after treatment ends. In the past, about 10% to 20% of men reported bowel problems after external beam radiation therapy, but the newer conformal radiation techniques may be less likely to cause these problems. I had none of these symptoms.

- **Bladder problems:** You might find yourself needing to urinate more often, having a burning sensation while you urinate, and finding blood in your urine. Bladder problems usually improve over time, but in some patients they never go away. About 1 patient out of 3 continues to have problems with needing to urinate more often. I also had none of these symptoms.

- **Urinary incontinence:** This side effect is less common than after surgery overall, but the chance of incontinence goes up each year for several years after treatment. No incontinence problems for me.

- **Impotence:** After a few years, the impotence rate after radiation is about the same as that of surgery. It usually does not occur right after radiation therapy but slowly develops over a year or more. This is different from surgery, where impotence occurs immediately and may improve over time. In older studies, about 3 out of 4 men were impotent within 5 years of having external beam radiation therapy (some of these men had erection problems before treatment). In men who had normal erections before treatment, about half became impotent at 5 years. It's not clear if these numbers will apply to newer forms of radiation as well. As with surgery, the older you are, the more likely it is you will become impotent. Impotence may be helped by treatments such as those listed in the section above, including erectile dysfunction medicines. This symptom was probably exacerbated by the Zoladex treatment as I am still impotent after stopping the Zoladex in 2006. However, I am starting to feel my libido again. So look out Rosie.

- **Feeling tired:** Radiation therapy may also cause fatigue that may not disappear until a few months after treatment stops. I don't recall feeling any more tired than usual.

I was feeling pretty fortunate that all but a one of the side effects that I was supposed to experience never materialized.

I had a chance to talk with several men going through the same procedure and asked them about the side effects they were experiencing. Like I said I feel fortunate. Several guys were experiencing almost all the symptoms, but a few were like me, just a limp willy.

According to Johns Hopkins [13], in a trial of short-term androgen-deprivation therapy, the Radiation Therapy Oncology Group (RTOG) treated 456 patients with external-beam radiation therapy alone or external-beam radiation therapy plus four months of androgen-deprivation therapy (beginning two months before external-beam radiation therapy and continuing for two months during EBRT). The men received goserelin (Zoladex) every four weeks and flutamide (Eulexin) three times daily before and during radiation treatment.

At 10 years, the overall survival rate was 43% for men receiving the combination therapy versus 34% for those treated with external-beam radiation therapy alone. Five years after treatment, 40% of the men treated with external-beam radiation therapy alone had developed bone metastases; in contrast, it took 13 years for 40% of the men in the combination group to develop them. In addition, at 10 years, 36% of the external-beam radiation therapy only group had died of prostate cancer compared with 23% of those treated with external-beam radiation therapy and androgen-deprivation therapy.

Bottom line: This study provides long-term confirmation that short-term androgen-deprivation therapy is beneficial in patients with high-risk, locally advanced disease who are undergoing external-beam radiation therapy.

Adding androgen-deprivation therapy to external-beam radiation therapy for a short period of time in men with locally advanced prostate cancer slows the rate of metastasis and improves disease-free survival, according to results from a decade-long study, reported in the *Journal of Oncology* (Volume 26, page 585).

Two months into my treatment a friend of mine couldn't sleep so he went downstairs to watch TV. When he turned on the set there was an infomercial on by Dr. Lorraine Day [7], who had beaten breast cancer by becoming a vegan [8]. That's not someone from the planet Vega nor is it a relative of our favorite Vulcan, Mr. Spock. The word "veganism" denotes a philosophy and way of living which seeks to exclude — as far as is possible and practical — all forms of exploitation of, and cruelty to, animals for food, clothing or any other purpose; and by extension, promotes the development and use of animal-free alternatives for the benefit of humans, animals and the environment. In dietary terms it denotes the practice of *dispensing with all products derived wholly or partly from animals*. My friend ordered her VHS tape and sent it to me. You can now get this in DVD format as well. After watching it I said, "I can do that!" Now a lot of people blast me because I still wear leather; shoes, belts etc. I explain to them that I am not doing this for moral reasons, but for health reasons.

Dr. Day was diagnosed with invasive breast cancer but rejected standard therapies because of their destructive side effects and because those therapies often lead to death. She chose instead to rebuild her immune system using the natural, simple, inexpensive therapies designed by God and outlined in the Bible, so her body could heal itself. When she found the lump in her breast she went to her oncologist friend at San Francisco General, he recommended a biopsy. She said absolutely not; cut the lump out and then biopsy it. She relayed to him that performing a biopsy on her would mean dragging possible cancer cells through healthy tissue thus spreading the cancer. After it was determined that she indeed had breast cancer he recommended chemotherapy and once again she said no, that chemo only caused another form of cancer. She would find an alternative cure. She found it in the bible. Adam and Eve did not eat flesh or any thing that came from the animals in the Garden of Eden. They ate what grew there, fruits, vegetables, nuts etc. Well the fruit thing was a bad idea.

Dr. Day deteriorated to the point her husband called in a priest to give her the last rites. Her cancer tumor and you will see this on the DVD, stuck out of her chest as if someone had rammed a baseball bat through her back. Her husband had to carry her everywhere in the house, bath her, and feed her. But, in 18 months after she had received the last rites and had started eating and practicing her new philosophy she was cancer free. The tumor had shrunk to nothing.

Dr. Day is an internationally acclaimed trauma surgeon and bestselling author who was for fifteen years on the faculty of the University of California, San Francisco, School of Medicine as Professor and Vice Chairman of the Department of Orthopedics. She was also Chief of Orthopedic Surgery at San Francisco General Hospital and is recognized world-wide as an AIDS expert.

She has been invited to lecture extensively throughout the U.S. and the world and has appeared on numerous radio and television shows including 60 Minutes, Nightline, CNN Crossfire, Oprah Winfrey, Larry king Live, The 700 Club, The John Ankerberg Show, USA Radio Network, Art Bell Radio Show, Three Angels Broadcasting Network and Trinity Broadcasting Network.

You can read all about Dr. Day at her web site, http://www.drday.com/. I highly recommend you purchase her DVD "Cancer Doesn't Scare Me Anymore", and follow her lead.

Six months after starting my hormone therapy, becoming a vegan and after going through 8 weeks of radiation therapy, I went back for my first check-up. The week before I went and had blood drawn for another PSA check. This was the first time that my doctor scared me, not intentionally. He came into the room and introduced himself and I said yes we had already met, several times... he sees a lot of people. "Maybe if I dropped my pants and bend over you'll recognize me... he didn't laugh. OK, so all Jews don't have sense of humor. He got on the computer to check for the results of my last PSA test and to see what my score was now. He is a soft spoken man and when he blurted out, "Holy Shit!" Well, it scared me. "What's wrong?" I demanded to know with some trepidation as I did and yet did not want to know what the bad news was. He asked, "Do you know what your PSA is?" I was thinking it had jumped to some astronomical number the way he had said "Holy shit!" "No, I don't." ".01" He said. Only the Lord and the laundry knew how bad he had scared me. He wanted to know if I had been doing anything that may have caused my score to drop so dramatically. At first I couldn't think of anything, but then I said, "Well, I became a vegan." He looked at me and said "Really! I'm going to tell all my patients to do consider this." Each subsequent check-up showed the same PSA... 0.01. So after three years of hormone therapy, January 2006, I said I wanted off as the hot flashes were just miserable and we could do the wait and see method. He said, "OK, I can live with that". Bad choice of words doc, I know you can, but can I.

Chapter 5

Sometime in 2008 my scores started to creep up, nothing dramatic, but by the end of 2009 my score had reached .20. Still way below what someone without cancer would even display, 1.5 to 3.5 is normal.

Another misadventure occurred during the time I was diagnosed and now. In January of 2004 the same good friend who had sent me Dr. Day's VHS asked if I would be interested in getting involved in a commercial realty software business. It is a software program that analyzes commercial real estate and determines in minutes as opposed to hours, days or months what a commercial property is really worth. Well I was pretty burned out with my beauty supply business after 25 years and the money sounded good. So I jumped in telling all my customers that they could come to my warehouse and get product at cost to eliminate my inventory... didn't happen. In 2006 I did a cash-out refinance of my house and put $180,000 into the company. This was bad timing as the RE market started its mighty plunge that is still felt today. Because commercial property was not selling neither was our software and we ran out of money ergo income for all of us and I lost my house.

The circumstance beyond my control mentioned previously was the move from my house after foreclosure to my mother's house. This was depressing to say the least... moving in with mommy at 70. I had been trying to put in a garden at my house for several years to no avail as the soil was mostly clay. I couldn't even grow dirt. I wanted to be able to grow vegetables and fruit that were definitely organic. You know what, God really DOES move in mysterious ways. My mother lives in Oxnard CA, a very large farming community and the soil is perfect. So I proceeded to dig up her back yard and plant a garden. So far I have been harvesting chard, mustard greens, corn, 5 varieties of tomatoes, red potatoes, 2 varieties of spinach, celery, 3 types of melons, 3 types of squash, 3 types of cabbage, Brussels sprouts, 2 varieties of cucumbers, red lettuce, romaine, four types of onions, oranges, lemons and a Ngami Kumquat tree.

My garden produces so much that I have been giving it away to my mother's caregivers, my sisters and cousins. If you can't grow your own garden then by all means find a local farmers market and buy your produce there. The foods we get from our supermarkets are loaded with chemicals and are nutritionally deficient.

After the Second World War, munitions manufacturers went to the government and asked for their help in keeping their doors open. One of the ingredients in making gunpowder is potassium nitrate, which is also used in fertilizers, NPK (nitrogen-phosphorus-potassium). Our government in all its wisdom went to the farmers and told them if they would use NPK they could grow more bountiful crops and that the government would give them a tax break and if not then the farmers would be summarily forced out of business. So, NPK it was. They were also informed that they would no longer have to rotate their crops, potatoes one year and corn the next. Farmers have known for generations that crop rotation avoids a decrease in soil fertility, as growing the same crop repeatedly in the same place eventually depletes the soil of various nutrients. A crop that leaches the soil of one kind of nutrient is followed during the next growing season by a dissimilar crop that returns that nutrient to the soil or draws a different ratio of nutrients, for example, rice followed by cotton. By crop rotation farmers can keep their fields under continuous production, without the need to let them lay fallow, and reducing the need for artificial fertilizers, both of which can be expensive.

Legumes, plants of the family Fabaceae, for instance, have nodules on their roots which contain nitrogen-fixing bacteria. It therefore makes good sense agriculturally to alternate them with cereals (family Poaceae) and other plants that require nitrates. A common modern crop rotation is alternating soybeans and maize (corn). In subsistence farming, it also makes good nutritional sense to grow beans and grain at the same time in different fields.

Those Enterprising chemical corporations, looking for a new market after World War II, developed NPK fertilizers in convenient granular form. But the soil was changing. The microscopic organisms and earthworms that had provided nutrients for native plants were either greatly reduced in numbers or completely eliminated by the new procedures. The soil became nearly devoid of life and essential trace elements depleted. There was also the problem of soil compaction and salt build-up.

Will farmers continue using NPK fertilizers ignoring soil biology until crops are lovely to look at but devoid of nutrition, and the land becomes useless, or will we, the consumer, force them to change? We, the consumer, are starting to make inroads in that direction by asking for organic foods, foods not sprayed with pesticides. As far as crop rotation, here in Oxnard, I still see the same crops planted in the same fields' season after season, strawberries predominately.

Christopher Zinn, from consumer magazine Choice, said of 27 samples of strawberries tested, three had higher than recommended MAX residue limits.

"The latest Choice test results clearly show the delectable strawberry as having far greater pesticide residue than any of the other 12 fruits and vegetables: peaches, nectarines, plums, apples, bell peppers, celery, cherries, grapes, potatoes, spinach and raspberries. Some are laced with banned chemicals," he said.

Of the conventionally grown strawberries tested bought from Coles, Woolworths/Safeway and independent fruit shops, a disturbing 11 per cent contained pesticide residues above the legal limit; 17 out of 27 samples, or 63 per cent, had residues of more than one pesticide; and four had four different pesticides.

"Strawberries, because of the kind of fruit they are, you eat their skin, they do tend to have a higher residue of pesticide on them," Zinn said.

Chapter 6

I purchased a Jack LaLanne Power Juicer Deluxe a few years ago and it is coming in very handy now. I juice fresh spinach, cucumber, celery, carrot and apple every morning mixing it with my colon cleanser. I've used many cleansers is the past, Metamucil, Citrucel, Serutan ("Natures spelled backwards.") was their advertising hook. It was what my maternal grandfather used. I was never really fond of any of them. I found a colon cleanser at my local Lassens health food store. It is a psyllium (cil-lium) whole husk all natural fiber supplement. You mix it with water or juice. I also have oatmeal every morning with raisins and dried cranberries, flax meal, raw almonds (about 10) and strawberries from the garden. Sometimes I sweeten it with raw honey. I also add rice milk, just a small amount to thin it out as the flax meal thickens it.

One great thing nowadays is that you can find more and more vegan products in places like Whole Foods and Trader Joes'. I get plenty of protein from beans, nuts and whole grains to name a few. Tofu and other soy foods are an excellent red meat alternative. But don't go overboard; 2 to 4 servings a week is a good target.

The Institute of Medicine recommends that adults get a minimum of 0.8 grams of protein for every kilogram of body weight per day—that's about 64 grams for a 160 pound adult. In the U.S., adults get an average of 15 percent of their calories from protein; for a person who requires a 2,000-calorie-per-day-diet, that's about 75 grams of protein. In healthy people, increasing protein intake to 20 to 25 percent of calories can reduce the risk of heart disease, if the extra protein replaces refined carbohydrates, such as white bread, white rice, or sugary drinks. Higher protein diets can also be beneficial for weight loss, in conjunction with a reduced calorie diet, although long-term evidence of their effectiveness is wanting. If you're going to eat red meat limit it to once a week or less. Forget chicken, too many hormones, unless you can find free range. But if you really want to fight that cancer… be a vegan.

Now something else I've done to fight my cancer. I've started drinking alkaline water. Cancer cannot live in an alkaline environment, this according to Dr. Theodore Baroody, in his book *Alkalize or Die.*

In 2010 I was introduced to alkaline water and told that research shows that cancer can't live in an alkaline environment. Just prior to my starting to drink alkaline water I went and had my PSA tested and my score was .21. Four months later after drinking approximately a gallon of alkaline water daily I went in for my quarterly PSA….20. It had dropped. OK, so .01 is not a big jump, but it is when it is going in the other direction. The machine that makes the alkaline water was too expensive for me and due to a circumstance beyond my control I was forced to reduce my water intake for 3 months. I finally decided to buy the machine on the layaway plan. The next month was my quarterly PSA, Yikes! .26. Still, that is very low as I said earlier. My doctor asked me, since I no longer see him but talk on the phone after every test result, if I had any weight loss, which can be a good indicator that the cancer has come back with a vengeance. "I wish" I said. "I'm still carrying the 20 lbs I gained while on the hormone therapy." "Good." He said. "We'll speak again in 4 months." Like the first PSA after starting my water program, I'm looking forward to my next test in 4 months to see if indeed my PSA has dropped.

Chapter 7

Vegan Cookbook

The internet is loaded with vegan recipes

Bulgur Stuffed Cabbage Rolls

1 Small cabbage
1 Cup parsley -- finely chopped
2 onions – chopped
4 Stalks celery – chopped
1/4 Tsp Italian seasoning
1/2 Tsp garlic – minced
30 oz tomato sauce
4 Cups water
2 Cups bulgur
8 oz tomato sauce

Remove core from cabbage, place cabbage head in steamer and steam until all leaves are soft and separate easily.

Sauté parsley, onions, celery, seasoning, and garlic in olive oil until onions are soft. Add 2 15-oz. cans of tomato sauce, 4 cups water and bulgur. Cook about 1/2 hr. over medium heat, stirring occasionally, until bulgur is tender. Remove from heat.

To stuff cabbage leaves, place a spoonful of mixture in center of each leaf. Starting at one side, roll leaf up and fold ends under. Place in a deep baking pan. Mix the 8 oz can of tomato sauce with 1/2 cup water and pour over stuffed cabbage leaves so they remain moist during baking. Bake at 375 for about 30 min. until cabbage is hot.

Cabbage Roll Casserole

2 pounds vegan ground beef (soy)
1 cup chopped onion
1 (29 ounce) can tomato sauce
3 1/2 pounds chopped cabbage
1 cup uncooked white rice
1 teaspoon salt
2 (14 ounce) cans vegetable broth

Preheat oven to 350 degrees F (175 degrees C).

In a large mixing bowl combine the onion, tomato sauce, cabbage, rice, salt and the soy ground beef... mix all together. Pour mixture into a 9x13 inch baking dish. Pour broth over mixture and bake in the preheated oven, covered, for 1 hour. Stir, replace cover and bake for another 30 minutes.

Mushroom Croustade

3oz flaked almonds
3oz whole wheat breadcrumbs
3oz ground almonds
1 small onion, peeled and grated
1 garlic clove, crushed
3½oz Smart Balance™
1lb mushrooms, washed and sliced
5fl oz soy cream
freshly grated nutmeg
paprika.

Preheat the oven to 350F

Reserve a few of the flaked almonds for garnishing. Mix together the breadcrumbs, ground and remaining flaked almonds, onion, garlic and 3oz of the Smart Balance™, season well with salt and pepper. The mixture should hold together like a crumbly pastry.

Press the mixture into the base of a 20cm/8 inch loose-bottomed flan tin. Bake for 20 minutes, until golden-brown and crisp.

Meanwhile, fry the mushrooms in the remaining Smart Balance™, for 15-20 minutes, until the liquid has evaporated, season with salt and pepper.

Spoon the mushrooms on top of the croustade. Season the soy cream with salt, pepper and nutmeg, and then swirl it on top of the mushrooms. Sprinkle with paprika.

Return the croustade to the oven for 10-15 minutes, to heat through, then remove from the tin and serve on a warmed plate. Scatter the reserved flaked almonds over the top.

Vegan Pancakes

12 oz of soy milk (sweetened or not)
3 heaped tbsp white self-rising flour
1 tsp soy flour
pinch of salt

Delicious sprinkled with sugar and lemon, or served with slices of fruit and vegan ice-cream. These also make a good savory dish filled with a bolognaise-style filling and topped with a vegan white sauce.

 Mix all the ingredients except the water in a blender and check the consistency by dipping a spoon into the mixture. It should evenly coat the back of the spoon. If necessary, add more soy milk or more flour.

Heat a heavy-bottomed or non-stick frying pan and pour in 1 teaspoon (no more) of vegetable oil. Ensure it evenly coats the pan.

Pour in ¼ of the mixture (this makes quite thick pancakes - use slightly less if you like them thinner). Tilt the pan quickly to ensure even coverage of the mixture. Cook on a medium heat until golden brown. Turn over and cook other side, then slide onto a plate and cook the next one.

Creamy Broccoli Soup

1 lb broccoli, chopped (approx 1 large one, stalk and florets)
2 tbsp vegetable oil
1 large leek, sliced
1 stick celery, chopped
½ green pepper, chopped
3 cloves garlic, chopped
1oz, chopped fresh ginger
1 bay leaf
24 ozs. water
1 tbsp lemon juice
pepper

Try adding more ginger (about half the quantity again) for a really tasty broccoli and ginger soup!

Gently fry the leek, celery, pepper, garlic, ginger and bay leaf in the oil for 10 minutes until the leek is soft.

Add the broccoli and water. Bring to the boil then simmer with the lid on for about 10 minutes.

Take the pan off the heat and leave the soup to cool a little. Remove the bay leaf and then blend the soup until smooth. Pour back into the pan and reheat. Add the pepper and lemon juice.

Serve with avocado wedges and multigrain crackers.

Cabbage Soup

2 32oz cartons of vegetable broth
2 14oz cans of Chinese sweet & sour sauce
1 head of cabbage
2 small zucchini chopped
1 med sweet onion chopped
2 carrots chopped
4-5 chard leaves ripped into bite size pieces
10 green beans chopped into ½ pieces
6 large asparagus spears chopped into ½ pieces
6 celery stalks chopped
6 brown mushrooms chopped
1 cup dried barley
1 cup dried black lentils
1 cup dried red lentils
3 small red potatoes cut into bite size pieces
Salt and pepper to taste

Add the broth and sauce to a large pot. Chop the cabbage in about inch pieces add to the pot and set temp to medium and bring to a boil. While waiting for the pot to boil start adding the rest of your ingredients, except the dried barley and lentils and potatoes. In another pot add the dried barley and lentils… rinse thoroughly, cover with water and cook per directions on the package. Once the veggies are tender and the barley and lentils are done mix together with the potatoes and cook until potatoes are tender. Salt and pepper to taste

I now get out my canning jars and using a canning funnel, fill the jars with the soup. Whatever is left over and isn't enough for a jar… dinner!

Cabbage Potato Soup

Preparation time: 20-30 minutes
serves 4-6
ingredients required:

2 tblsp Smart Balance ™
1 medium cooking onion/diced
4 cloves fresh garlic/chopped finely
3 large potatoes/diced
1 1/2 stalks of celery/chopped finely
1 1/2 cups of cabbage/sliced and chopped
4 cups of vegetable broth
1/2 cup soy milk
1 tblsp flour
1 cup tofu sour cream
1 tsp salt or to taste
1/2 tsp red chili pepper

Optional:
1/8 cup finely diced sweet red pepper or 12 strips for garnish

Sauté onion & garlic on low heat until soft and fragrant, add red pepper (chili) flakes, sauté an additional 1 minute. Add raw potatoes, celery, cabbage, broth & simmer 15 minutes.

Remove 2 cups of the vegetables from the pot and place in blender or food processor with soy milk, soy sour cream and flour, puree until smooth. Stir back into soup and reheat.

Minute Minestrone Soup

1 Tbsp. olive oil
2 cloves garlic, minced
1 small onion, chopped
1 carrot, grated
2 small zucchini, diced
2 cups cabbage, shredded

2 cups vegetable broth
1 15-oz. can diced tomatoes
1 15-oz. can cannelloni beans, drained
1 tsp. dried rosemary

Sauté the onions and garlic in the olive oil till soft. Add rest of vegetables and continue sautéing till soft. Add the broth, tomatoes and beans into a large pot; bring to a boil and reduce heat to simmer adding the vegetable mix. Simmer until hot. Add dried rosemary let sit for 15 minutes and serve. Serve with vegan garlic bread.

Skinny (Cabbage) Soup

6 large green onions
2 bell peppers
1 or 2 large cans of tomatoes
1 bunch of celery
1 head of cabbage
1 package of Lipton onion soup mix
bouillon (optional)

Season with salt, pepper, curry, parsley, etc. if desired

Cut the vegetables into small pieces & cover with water. Boil fast for ten minutes.

Cut to a simmer and continue cooking vegetables until tender.

This soup can be eaten anytime you are hungry. Eat as much as you want, whenever you want, and at anytime of the day. This soup will not add calories.

Ginger-scented Tomato & Cabbage Soup

Yield: 4 servings

1/2 cup Alphabet spaghetti
2 med Onions, coarsely chopped
5 ea Garlic cloves, chopped
2 tbs Olive oil
1 smalll Carrot, diced
2 tsp Ginger, grated
2 cup Tomatoes, diced
6 cup Stock
1/2 ea Cabbage, thinly sliced
15 ea Fresh mint leaves, sliced
Salt & pepper
Cayenne

Cook pasta until al dente. Drain & set aside.

Lightly sauté onion & garlic in olive oil until softened. Stir in ginger & carrot & cook for a few moments. Add tomatoes, stock & cabbage.

Cook over medium heat until the vegetables are tender, 15 to 20 minutes. Adjust seasonings if necessary.

Ladle soup over several spoonfuls of cooked pasta. Season with fresh mint & serve immediately.

Vegan Creamed Spinach

Fresh, citrusy and light, this creamed spinach pairs perfectly with lighter fare or cool weather entrées.

Ingredients:
12 cups fresh baby spinach
1 cup plain gluten-free soymilk, unsweetened
2 teaspoons orange zest, finely grated
2 teaspoons lemon zest, finely grated
2 teaspoons vegan margarine
1/2 cup yellow onion, minced
Pinch of nutmeg
Sea salt, to taste
4 tablespoons sliced almonds, toasted

Method:
Steam spinach with a few tablespoons of water until just wilted. Squeeze out excess water and coarsely chop.

Place soymilk, orange zest and lemon zest in a small saucepan and bring to a boil. Simmer stirring frequently until reduced by half.

Heat margarine over medium heat in sauté pan and add onion. Cook until onion is translucent. Add spinach and cook until most of liquid has evaporated.

Add reduced soymilk to spinach and cook until thickened, stirring occasionally. Season with a pinch of nutmeg and sea salt to taste. Garnish with sliced almonds.

Vegan Broccoli Salad

3/4 cup Follow Your Heart™ Veganaise
1/4 cup red wine vinegar
2 tbsp Organic Blue Agave Sweetener
approx 2 cups broccoli, chopped
¼ cup red onion, finely chopped
½ cup cashews
¼ cup pinenuts
1 cup raisins
soy bacon bits
salt and pepper, to taste

In a small bowl, mix together the veganaise, vinegar and agave sweetener and set aside (this is your dressing).

In a separate large bowl, combine the broccoli, raisins and cashews.

Pour the dressing over the broccoli. Add a sprinkle of salt and pepper, to taste.

Vegan Coleslaw

1 head of organic cabbage
3 organic carrots
1 cup Follow Your Heart Vegenaise
1 tablespoon red wine vinegar
2 tablespoons fresh organic lemon juice
1 tablespoon fresh organic tangerine juice
1 ½ tablespoons caraway seeds
½ cup raisins
½ cup dried cranberries
1 tsp Tajin™ seasoning (You'll find this in the Mexican food section)

Shred your cabbage and carrots and mix well together. Add the Vegenaise and mix well, start with ½ cup and add small amounts until mixture is well coated. Add remaining ingredients and mix well. Place in a lidded container and store in refrigerator for 24 hours before serving. Most slaws have sugar added to offset the cabbage. If you want to fight cancer... stay away from sugar.

Chinese Cabbage Salad

1 (3 ounce) package ramen noodles, crushed
10 ounces cashew pieces
1 (16 ounce) bag of cabbage coleslaw
1 bunch green onions, chopped
1/2 cup white sugar
1/2 cup vegetable oil
1/4 cup cider vinegar
1 tablespoon soy sauce

In a preheated 350 degree F oven (175 degree C), toast the crushed noodles and nuts until golden brown.
In a large bowl, combine the coleslaw, green onions, toasted ramen noodles and cashews.
To prepare the dressing, whisk together the sugar, oil, vinegar and soy sauce. Pour the dressing over the salad, toss and serve.

Cabbage & Sweet-Corn Salad

1/2 of a hard white cabbage finely shredded
1 can of sweet-corn
3 tsp of Follow Your Heart Veganaise ™
A little salt. Mix everything together.

Vegan Greek Salad

2 tbsp olive oil
splash cider vinegar
½ tsp salt
1 tsp oregano
2 ripe tomatoes, cut into quarters, then cut the quarters in half
half a cucumber, cut into ½" slices, then cut the slices into quarters
2 thin slices onion, chopped small
freshly ground black pepper
10 black kalamata olives

Mix the ingredients together and leave to stand for half an hour.
Heat olive oil in a large saucepan and sauté garlic, onion, carrot and zucchini until tender.
Add cabbage and continue cooking until cabbage is tender.
Add remaining ingredients and cook over medium heat for 15 - 20 minutes.

Vegan White Sauce

2 oz Smart Balance™
1½ oz plain flour
14 oz. Soy milk

For a cheese flavor, 1 to 2 tbsp nutritional yeast flakes, to taste.

Put all the ingredients in a saucepan and whisk over the heat until cooked, season with freshly ground black pepper.

This is delicious served with steamed cauliflower or braised leeks, or mixed with diced cooked beetroot or fried onions, or use with bolognaise sauce in a vegan lasagna.

Vegan Gravy

Sometimes you like a little gravy on your mashed potatoes. This one is excellent.

1 onion, diced
2 tbsp oil
2 tbsp plain flour
clove of garlic (crushed)
15 fl oz vegetable stock
1 tsp yeast extract
1 or 2 tbsp soya sauce
freshly ground black pepper

As a variation, try adding a diced red pepper, a handful of cashew nuts, about 8 diced button mushrooms and a dash of red wine vinegar. Rather than straining the gravy, whizz it in a blender.

Fry the onion in the oil for 5 minutes.

Add the flour and cook for a further 5 to 10 minutes until the flour and onion are nut-brown and the onion is soft and slightly pulpy.

Add the garlic then gradually stir in the vegetable stock (or the water from any vegetables you happen to be boiling at the same time). Bring to the boil and simmer for 10 minutes.

Add the yeast extract, soya sauce and black pepper. Stir well. Strain if you like, or serve as it is.

Marinara Sauce

1 28oz can of chopped tomatoes
1 28oz can of tomato sauce
1 6oz can tomato paste
1 can med pitted olives
5 mushrooms sliced thin
1 soy Italian sausage
½ cup chopped Italian parsley
½ cup fresh basil chopped
Italian seasoning
Salt and pepper to taste

The big pot you used for the soup, get it out again or if you like to use a crock pot go for it. Add all the ingredients, but not the salt and pepper... you may not need it. If you're using your crock pot, set it on med and let it simmer for about 6 hours. If you use a regular stainless steel pot then bring to a boil, reduce the heat and simmer stirring occasionally. Keep an eye on it however; it may want to stick to the bottom of the pot, if you have thin bottomed pot. I do the same with this recipe as the soup... I can it.

Vegan Worcestershire Sauce

1/2 cup apple cider vinegar
2 tablespoons soy sauce
2 tablespoons water
1 tablespoon brown sugar
1/4 teaspoon ground ginger
1/4 teaspoon dry mustard
1/4 teaspoon onion powder
1/4 teaspoon garlic powder
1/8 teaspoon cinnamon
1/8 teaspoon pepper

Place all ingredients in a medium saucepan and stir thoroughly. Bring to a boil, stirring constantly. Simmer 1 minute. Cool.

Store in the refrigerator, makes about 3/4 cups.

Vegan Bolognaise Sauce

1 tbsp olive oil
1 onion, diced
1 stick celery, finely chopped
2 cloves garlic, chopped
¼ lb mushrooms, diced small
1 tin plum tomatoes
soya sauce
vegan Worcestershire sauce (See below)
1 tbsp tomato purée
2 tsp mixed herbs
1 tsp oregano
paprika

Use this recipe with some vegan white sauce for a tasty vegan lasagna. Serve with garlic bread (made with vegan margarine) and salad.

Fry the onion in the oil until it starts to brown. Add the celery and garlic and stir well.

Add the mushrooms and a dash of soya sauce and vegan Worcestershire sauce **(standard Worcestershire sauce contains anchovies)**. Cook for a few minutes and then the tomatoes, around 150ml water, the herbs, a pinch of paprika and the tomato puree. Simmer away for 10 to 15 minutes.

In the meantime cook some spaghetti, and when it is ready toss it in some Smart Balance™, pile the vegan bolognaise sauce on top and add some freshly ground black pepper.

Spicy Bean Burgers

1 carrot, diced small
2 tbsp oil
1 onion, chopped small
1 clove garlic, chopped
1 tsp ground cumin
1 tsp ground coriander
1 tsp dried mixed herbs
½ tsp paprika
½ tsp chilli powder
4 oz cooked red kidney beans (half a 400g tin, rinsed and drained)
4 oz cooked chick peas (ditto)
1 tbsp cooked sweet-corn
1 level tbsp flour

Boil the carrot until al dente then drain.

Meanwhile, heat 1 tbsp of the oil in a frying pan and fry the onion and garlic for 5 minutes until soft and starting to brown.

Add the herbs, spices and flour, and cook for 1 min, stirring well (don't let the flour burn).

Mash the beans and chick peas with a fork. Mix in the onion mixture, the carrots and sweet corn and mash some more, season to taste.

Heat the remaining oil, shape the mixture into 4 burgers and fry for 5 to 6 minutes on each side till done. Delicious!

Vegan Garden Burger

2 tbsp pecan nuts
¾ cup fresh breadcrumbs
vegetable oil for sautéing
1 small onion
2 cloves garlic
½ red or orange (sweet bell) pepper
8oz mushrooms
1 mild or hot chilli (optional)
1 tbsp hoisin sauce
½ cup cooked rice (1/3 cup before cooking)
salt & black pepper to taste
2 tbsp potato flakes to help bind (optional)

First, toast and grind the pecan nuts. Cook them in a dry frying pan over a low heat for about 5 minutes, stirring often, until slightly browned but not burned. Grind in a blender or food processor - it helps to add some of the breadcrumbs to the blender to stop the nuts flying all over the place.

Chop the onion and garlic, sauté in vegetable stock (or oil if you prefer) until softened and slightly browned.

Meanwhile, chop the pepper and mushrooms. Finely chop the chilli (if using). When the onions are ready, add these other vegetables and cook for a further 10-15 minutes until everything is tender, adding a little water if things start to stick.

Add the hoisin sauce, mix well and continue to cook until the sauce is thick.

Place the vegetable mixture in a blender along with the cooked rice, and pulse a few times to blend things together, leaving some pieces of vegetables whole.

Mix in the toasted, ground pecan nuts and breadcrumbs, season to taste only if necessary. If the mixture seems a bit sloppy, mix in some potato flakes or instant mashed potato to help bind it. Don't use flour as it won't have time to cook properly.

If possible, leave in the fridge to firm up for 30 minutes - it will keep there for a few days. Form into burgers - you can make them quite thin and flat, with smooth edges. To cook them, fry or bake. Be careful when turning them not to disturb the browned crust.

Vegan BLT

1 large white roll
Smart Balance™
Follow Your Heart™ Veganaise
tomato relish
wholegrain mustard
ketchup
vegan bacon (see recipe below)
tomato, sliced
lettuce, shredded

Find the largest white roll you possibly can. Spread generously with the Smart Balance™ then the veganaise and all the relishes.

Fry the vegan bacon to desired crispiness and place in roll.

Add slices of tomato and some fresh, crisp lettuce to your BLT and enjoy!

Vegan Bacon

tempeh
soy sauce
sunflower oil
salt and pepper

Slice the tempeh, and marinate in soy sauce for an hour or more. Fry in a little hot oil, turning once.

Garlicky Mustard Greens

3 pounds mustard greens
1 tablespoon olive oil
1 cup chopped onions
3 cloves garlic
1 large red bell pepper, chopped (about one cup)
1/2 cup chicken broth, canned or homemade
1 tablespoon cider vinegar
2 teaspoons sugar

Pick through the greens removing yellow, wilted greens and large tough stems and veins. Run the sink full of cool water and wash the greens in three changes of water. Fresh greens hold soil and dirt. Swishing the greens through the cold water removes grit the clinging grit. Drain. Stack several leaves; roll up jelly-roll style. Cut crosswise into 1/2 inch slices. Repeat with remaining greens. Heat oil in Dutch oven or large saucepan over medium heat, add onion and garlic, cook and stir for about 3 minutes. Stir in greens, red bell pepper and chicken broth. Bring to boil then reduce heat to low. Cook, covered for 20 to 25 minutes or until greens are tender. Young greens cook quickly; large older greens can take as long as 45 minutes to become tender. Add more water if needed. In a small bowl, combine vinegar and sugar. Stir until dissolved. Sprinkle over cooked greens, remove from heat. Serve immediately.

Makes 6 servings

Cinnamon-Glazed Baby Carrots

4 cups baby carrots
2 tablespoons Smart Balance™ Margarine
2 tablespoons organic brown sugar
½ teaspoon organic ground cinnamon
1/8 teaspoon salt

1. Place carrots in a small sauce pan. Add just enough of water to barely cover the carrots. Cover and bring to a boil. Reduce heat to medium. Cook for 7 to 8 minutes, just until carrots are easily pierced with a sharp knife.
2. Combine margarine, brown sugar, cinnamon and salt in a small saucepan, and melt together over low heat. Stir well to combine ingredients.
3. Drain carrots, leading them in a saucepan. Pour cinnamon mixture over carrots. Cook and stir over medium heat for 2-3 minutes, just until the carrots are thoroughly coated and the glaze thickens slightly. Serve warm.

Serves about 4

Vegan Potato Salad

2 medium russet or rose potatoes
1/3 cup Veganaise
2 tablespoons mustard (vary the type each time)
juice of ½ lime
6 -7 black olives chopped
6 -7 pimento stuffed olives chopped
2 - 3 tablespoons kosher dill pickles chopped

- Peel and chop potatoes into ½" cubes, steam. Put steamed potatoes into refrigerator to cool, about 1 hour or more. Add rest of ingredients and mix till well coated. Place in a container and put in regrigerator.

Sweet Potato Salad

4 small sweet potatoes
¼ cup Veganaise
1 tablespoon mustard
4 celery stalks, sliced ¼ inch thick
1 small red bell pepper, cut into quarter inch dice
1 cup diced fresh pineapple
2 scallions, finely chopped
salt and pepper
½ cup coarsely chopped toasted pecans
chopped fresh chives

1. Preheat oven to 400° F. Wrap each sweet potato in foil and bake for 1 hour. Unwrap; let cool. Peel; cut into ¾ inch chunks.
2. In a large bowl, mix Veganaise and mustard. And sweet potatoes, celery, red pepper, pineapple, and the scallions; toss gently. Season to taste with salt and pepper. Cover and refrigerate about 1 hour.
3. Fold in pecans and sprinkle with chives.

Sweet Corn Pudding

2 large eggs (see vegan substitutes for eggs)
¾ cup evaporated milk (see vegan substitutes for evaporated milk)
2 cups canned cream style corn
2 cups fresh or frozen corn kernels
2 tablespoons unsalted margarine melted
3 tablespoons organic dark brown sugar
3 tablespoons cornstarch
1/2 teaspoon ground nutmeg
1/4 teaspoons salt
1/8 teaspoon ground white pepper

1. Prepare the oven to 330° F. Butter and 80 inch square baking dish.
2. Whisk together the eggs and milk. Stir in the remaining ingredients.
3. Pour the mixture into the banking dish. Bake 45 to 48 minutes, or until lightly browned. Serve will warm up

    Serves 8

No-Bake Cookies

Ingredients:

- 2 cups pitted dates
- 2 cup finely chopped almonds
- 1 cup coarse chopped almonds
- 1 cup shredded coconut
- ½ cup raisins
- ½ cup dried cranberries
- 1 tsp lemon juice
- 1 tsp nutmeg

Place all ingredients in a food processor except the finely chopped almonds. Blend until crumbly and sticking together.

Take a small golf ball sized amount of the mixture and roll in the palm of your hands until round. Place the finely chopped almonds in a dinner plate. Place the roll of mixture on the plate and push down forming a cookie. Coat the other side of the cookie with the finely chopped almonds and place on another plate. Once you have all the cookies on the other plate, cover with plastic wrap and place in the refrigerator. Serve in about 1-2 hours

Vegan Pie Crust

Use this vegan pie crust recipe for any pie, vegan or not

The secret to successful vegan pie crust is to chill every single ingredient, plus the pastry blender and the bowl. For best results, handle the dough with your hands as little as possible.

Makes enough for one single crust 9 inch pie, or a double crust pie
You'll have a bit of crust left over for a few tarts or pie crust cookies, invented by children for children (cut out shapes with cookie cutter, sprinkle with sugar and cinnamon

Ingredients - Single Crust:

- 1 1/2 cups all purpose flour
- 2/3 cup frozen Earth Balance veggie spread
- Ice water

Ingredients - Double Crust Pie:

- 2 1/2 cups all purpose flour
- 1 cup frozen Earth Balance veggie spread
- Ice water

Directions:

1. Chill flour and pastry blender in large mixing bowl for 1/2 an hour - the freezer is ideal
2. Cut the frozen veggie spread into the flour with a pastry blender or a fork until the mixture resembles a coarse meal
3. Rub together with your hands until the veg spread is absorbed into the flour and the mixture is crumbly (this prevents crumbly dough)
4. Add a few Tbsp ice water gradually, mixing with a fork, just until it starts to clump together

5. Handling the dough as little as possible, quickly form a ball of dough
6. Press the dough flat into a disk and roll out on a lightly floured surface with a lightly floured rolling pin
7. For the best results, roll away from your body and after every one or two strokes give the dough a slight clockwise turn. Lift the dough partway up and sprinkle more flour underneath as needed
8. Continue rolling and rotating until the crust is about 3 inches larger in diameter than the rim of the pie plate
9. Carefully transfer the crust to the pie plate by folding the dough in half and quickly lifting it to the pie plate and then unfolding it
10. Center the crust and trim so that the crust hangs slightly over the edge
11. Flute the edges by placing the thumb on the outer side of the crust and the two index fingers on either side of the thumb in the inside of the crust. Push the thumb forward while pulling the index fingers toward you
12. Continue clockwise in this manner until you have gone all way around the rim of the pie
13. For a double crust add the filling and the top crust before trimming and fluting
14. Slash 3 steam vents in the top crust in a spoke pattern or just make a large 'V' if your pie will be served alongside non-vegan pies

Whipped Coconut Cream

Ingredients:

- 1 1/2 cups full fat coconut milk, from two 13.5 oz cans
- 1/3 cup powdered sugar or to taste
- 1 - 4 Tbsp coconut flour or tapioca flour (add 1 Tbsp at a time)
- 1 Tbsp vanilla extract or to taste

Directions:

1. Open the cans of coconut milk, transfer to a glass or metal bowl using a rubber spatula
2. Cover with a lid, plate, or plastic wrap and refrigerate at least 4 hours, or overnight
3. Beat the thick coconut cream in the chilled bowl with a hand mixer until thick and fluffy
4. Gradually beat in the powdered sugar and coconut or tapioca flour, 1 or 2 Tbsp at a time, testing for flavor and consistency
5. For flavored whipped cream, add some cinnamon, instant coffee, or cocoa powder (you may want to increase the sugar a bit); or replace the vanilla with almond or coconut extract or a liqueur
6. Using a rubber spatula, transfer the coconut cream to a covered storage container, and refrigerate until needed

Whipped Cashew Cream

Ingredients:

- 1 cup raw cashews
- 2 cups filtered white grape, pear or apple juice
- 2 Tbsp sunflower seed oil, or melted coconut oil
- 1/4 cup powdered sugar or to taste
- 1 tsp vanilla or to taste

Directions:

1. Bring the cashews and juice to a boil, then reduce heat and simmer until the cashews soften (5 - 10 minutes)
2. Cover, and leave to cool for a couple of hours, or overnight in the fridge
3. Drain the cashews, reserving the liquid
4. Blend the cashews with the oil and vanilla, adding a small amount of the reserved juice as needed to help things along. Use as little liquid as possible - the cream should be thick
5. Add the sugar gradually, testing until it has the right amount sweetness for you
6. Using a rubber spatula, transfer the cream from the blender to a covered storage container, and refridgerate until needed

Vegan Apple Pie

Ingredients:

1. 8-10 medium large apples (enough to make 6 cups of apple slices)
2. 1/2 to 1 cup sugar (according to preference and sweetness of the apples. The tarter the apple, the greater the amount of sugar)
3. Optional: 1/4 - 1/2 tsp cinnamon
4. 1 1/2 Tbsp cornstarch
5. 1 Tbsp lemon juice
6. 1 double recipe Vegan Pie Crust

Directions:

1. Prepare pie crust, wrap tightly and chill for 1/2 - 1 hour (no more!)
2. Peel, quarter, and core the apples
3. Slice each quarter into thin even slices
4. Mix together the sugar, cinnamon, and cornstarch. Gently stir into apples until well coated. Stir in lemon juice
5. Preheat oven to 425 degrees F
6. Roll out top and bottom crusts, making the top one about 50% bigger
7. Place apples in bottom pie crust. Cover with top crust, flute edges together, and use a knife to make several steam vents
8. Bake at 450 for 10 minutes and then turn the oven down to 350. Continue baking for 35 to 45 minutes
9. The pie is done when the crust is golden and the contents are bubbling. Insert a fork gently into a steam vent to see if the apples are tender. If the crust is done but the apples are not, turn the oven down to 300 and bake another 10 or 15 minutes, until the apples are tender

Replacing Dairy in Vegetarian and Vegan Desserts

Milk: The best milk substitute for baking is soymilk with almond milk a close second. The reason they work so well is that they have fat, unlike rice milk. Rice milk is great when you are cooking, but using rice milk in baking will result in desserts that are dry and less than rich and satisfying.

1 cup soy or almond milk = 1 cup dairy milk

Buttermilk: Substitute an equal amount of soymilk mixed with lemon juice. Allow the mixture to thicken 5 minutes before using. Or substitute an equal amount of vegan sour cream substitute diluted half and half with water.

1 cup buttermilk = 1 cup soymilk with 2 Tblsp lemon juice allowed to sit 5 minutes

1 cup buttermilk = 1/2 cup vegan sour cream mixed with 1/2 cup water

Sour Cream: Use a vegan sour cream substitute. I've had good luck with Sour Supreme, when making things like vegan blueberry sour cream muffins.

1 cup sour cream = 1 cup vegan sour cream

1 Cup sour cream = 1 cup soy yogurt

Butter: Use a vegan butter substitute. My favorite is Earth Balance buttery spread. Because vegan butter substitutes tend to be less solid than dairy butter, make sure you freeze it before you use it in a vegan pie crust, and chill the crust 15 minutes before rolling it and again before baking it. That's if you want a tender, flaky pie crust! Also, unless you can find salt-free vegan butter, it's a good idea to reduce the salt in the recipe by half. Vegetable oil can also replace butter or vegetable spread in most recipes. Use around 25% less oil - 3/4 cup oil to 1 cup butter or veggie spread.

1 cup butter = 1 cup vegan butter = 3/4 cup vegetable oil

Cream: Coconut cream (the thick portion skimmed off the top of whole fat coconut milk) and tofu are non-dairy alternatives. Coconut cream can be used as a straight substitute for dairy cream in your favorite whipped cream recipe. Tofu offers versatility, based upon the type you purchase. Soft tofu will yield a light cream when pureed, while extra-firm tofu will produce your thickest option. For a truly creamy texture, always choose varieties that are labeled as 'Silken.' For pumpkin pies and cheesecakes, the non-silken tofu selections will give your dessert a more traditional texture.

Cheese: Replacing cream cheese and ricotta cheese in vegan baking.

Ricotta Cheese: Substitute an equal quantity of mashed soft or silken tofu blended with a dash of lemon juice.

Cream Cheese: Blend a dash of lemon juice with heavy coconut cream.

Replacing Eggs in Vegetarian and Vegan Desserts

Eggs have two functions in baking: Binding or thickening and leavening (leavening is what makes baked goods light and fluffy.) Identifying their function in a particular recipe will help you decide with how to replace them. Different egg replacers will work best in different recipes. Be prepared to do a little experimenting. Ener-G Egg Replacer will work well in most dishes. Ener-G Egg Replacer is designed for use in baking. It works best in scratch recipes. It will not make scrambled eggs. Although it will work well in some pre-made commercial mixes, it does not work well in others. Trial and error is the only way to determine its effectiveness with a particular mix. Egg replacer mimics what eggs do in a baking recipe. It is important to put the batter of dough quickly into a preheated oven to ensure proper action as a delay will reduce the effectiveness of this product. With yeast raised products there is no need to get products containing egg replacer into the oven quickly

In cookies and muffins, no binding agent is generally needed. In quick breads and cakes both leavening and binding is needed. In custard pies, like pumpkin pie, eggs are mainly for thickening. You won't be able to make really light types of desserts that call for a very large number of eggs, but you will be able to make just about anything else that uses up to 3-4 eggs.

Leavening: For cakes, cookies, muffins, quick breads, etc

Soymilk with lemon: 1 egg = 1/4 cup soymilk + 1 Tblsp lemon

Sour Supreme and baking soda: 1 egg = 1/4 cup Sour Supreme + 1/4 tsp baking soda

Optional: In cakes and quick breads, add 2 Tblsp of cornstarch to the dry ingredients for each egg being replaced. This will bind the ingredients and give a nice soft texture.

Thickening and Binding:

Finely ground flaxseeds whipped with water: 1 egg = 1 Tblsp ground flax seeds mixed with 1/4 cup water

The flaxseeds gel and bind with the other ingredients. Some people find that this works best with a little Ener G Egg replacer mixed in since flax seeds alone have no leavening effect.

Cornstarch and pureed soft tofu: 1 egg = 3 Tblsp pureed tofu + 2 tsp cornstarch (Good for quiches and custard pies.)

Optional: In cakes and quick breads, add 2 Tblsp of cornstarch to the dry ingredients for each egg being replaced. This will bind the ingredients and give a nice soft texture.

Commercial Egg Replacers: Also a good all-purpose egg substitute, but some people find that it leaves a bitter aftertaste.

Fat Free Egg Replacers: 1/4 cup applesauce, pureed banana, squash or pumpkin, will also work as egg replacers for binding. They are low in fat but will also add some flavor, which may or may not be desirable depending on the recipe.

1 egg = 1/4 cup puree

Ready Made Dessert Toppers: Look for Turtle Mountain's Purely Decadent and Soy Delicious lines, available in most supermarkets in North America (even Walmart). For a good non-soy dessert topper, Good Karma's Organic Rice Divine™ can be found at Trader Joe's and other natural food retailers. Whole Soy Co. offers a deliciously creamy, low fat line of soy frozen yogurts. Soyatoo (in spray cans) is a soy based whipped cream substitute. Luna & Larry's Coconut Bliss ice creams are rich, calorie laden and taste divine with fruit pie or crisp

Now that you know how to make all your favorite desserts into vegan delights, get baking!

Vegan Pumpkin Pie

Pumpkin pie made with fresh pumpkin is in a whole different taste universe than pumpkin pie made with canned pumpkin.

Cooking Tips: One 5 lb pie pumpkin is usually enough for two pies, and you can also use butternut squash. But if you are pressed for time, of course its okay to use canned. Pumpkin pie fans won't mind, but you won't make any converts!

Use your own pie crust recipe, buy a ready-made crust, or try our no-fail vegan pie crust. For two pumpkin pies, double the pie filling recipe.

Nutrition Info for 1 Serving, 120 g: 158 calories, 28g carbohydrate, 5g fat, 12mg sodium, 1g dietary fiber, 2g protein, Estimated glycemic load: 18 This food is very low in Cholesterol and Sodium. It is also a good source of Manganese, and a very good source of Vitamin A

6 - 8 servings: This recipe makes one 9" vegan pumpkin pie. It's lovely by itself, and *fabulous* with coconut whipped cream or cashew cream.

Pie Filling Ingredients:

- 1 unbaked single vegan pie crust
- 2 cups fresh cooked puréed pumpkin or butternut squash - see directions below. (Or one 16 oz can)
- 3/4 cup full fat coconut milk
- 1/3 cup soft silken tofu
- 2 Tbsp all purpose flour
- 1 tsp vanilla
- 1 tsp cinnamon
- 1 tsp ginger
- 1/2 tsp nutmeg
- 2 Tbsp light organic molasses (NOT blackstrap - too strong)
- 1/2 c. organic unbleached cane sugar OR brown sugar
- 2 Tbsp Ener-G egg replacer

Pie Filling Directions:

1. Preheat oven to 425 degrees
2. Blend all ingredients in a blender or food processor
3. Pour the pie filling into the unbaked pie crust (dust with flour first)
4. Bake at 425 for 10 minutes, then reduce heat to 350 and cook for 30 more minutes until the pie is almost completely firm in the center and the crust is golden. It will be slightly jiggley in the center
5. Remove from oven and cool completely before serving

Cooking Pumpkin or Squash:

1. One 3 - 4 lb pie pumpkin, or butternut squash
2. Using a big sharp knife, cut into 8 pieces & remove seed pulp
3. Place in a large baking pan, filled with 1/4 inch of water, and cover with foil or a tight fitting lid
4. Bake at 350 degrees for 1 hour, or until tender
5. Let cool, covered, then scoop the pumpkin out of the skins
6. Puree in a food processor, blender, or put through a sieve or food mill
7. Refrigerate or freeze what you don't need for pumpkin bread or pumpkin soup

References

[1] Page 1
http://www.johnshopkinshealthalerts.com/alerts/prostate_disorders/J
ohnsHopkinsProstateDisordersHealthAlert_3423-
1.html?ET=johnshopkins_blog:e37501:938758a:&st=email&st=ema
il&s=EPH_100428_005

[2] Page 2 http://www.usana.com/dotCom/about/founder

[3] Page 4 http://men.webmd.com/prostate-biopsy

[4] Page 4 http://www.prostate-
cancer.org/education/staging/Dowd_GleasonScore.html

[5] Page 5 http://www.healthsquare.com/newrx/zol1502.htm

[6] http://www.cancer.gov/cancertopics/factsheet/Risk/vasectomy

[7]
http://www.cancer.org/docroot/cri/content/cri_2_4_4x_androgen_su
ppression_hormone_therapy_36.asp

[8] http://www.webmd.com/hw-popup/bone-scan-of-the-spread-of-
prostate-cancer

[9]
http://www.cancer.org/docroot/CRI/content/CRI_2_4_4X_Radiation
_Therapy_36.asp

[10] http://www.drday.com/

[11] http://en.wikipedia.org/wiki/Veganism

[12]
http://www.johnshopkinshealthalerts.com/alerts/prostate_disorders/J
ohnsHopkinsHealthAlertsProstateDisorders_2237-1.html

[13]
http://www.johnshopkinshealthalerts.com/alerts/prostate_disorders/johnsH
opkinsProstateDisordersHealthAlert_3427-

1.html?ET=johnshopkins_blog:e39091:938758a:&st=email&st=email&s=
EPH_100609_005

www.ingramcontent.com/pod-product-compliance
Lightning Source LLC
Chambersburg PA
CBHW060217290526
45789CB00003B/1299